AF720307

ESSENTIAL LIFE SKILLS

MANAGING YOUR HEALTH AND WELL-BEING

by Andy Minshew

BrightPoint Press

San Diego, CA

BrightPoint Press

© 2027 BrightPoint Press
an imprint of ReferencePoint Press, Inc.
Printed in the United States

For more information, contact:
BrightPoint Press
PO Box 27779
San Diego, CA 92198
www.BrightPointPress.com

ALL RIGHTS RESERVED.
No part of this work covered by the copyright hereon may be reproduced or used in any form or by any means—graphic, electronic, or mechanical, including photocopying, recording, taping, web distribution, or information storage retrieval systems—without the written permission of the publisher. No part of this book may be used or reproduced in any manner for the purpose of training artificial intelligence technologies or systems.

LIBRARY OF CONGRESS CATALOGING-IN-PUBLICATION DATA

Names: Minshew, Andy, author.
Title: Managing your health and well-being / by Andy Minshew.
Description: San Diego, CA: ReferencePoint Press, [2027] | Series: Essential life skills | Includes bibliographical references and index. | Audience term: Teenagers | Audience term: Children | Audience: Grades 7–9
Identifiers: LCCN 2026007262 (print) | LCCN 2026007263 (eBook) | ISBN 9781678214548 hardcover | ISBN 9781678214555 eBook
Subjects: LCSH: Teenagers--Health and hygiene | Youth--Health and hygiene | Well-being
Classification: LCC RA564.5 .M56 2027 (print) | LCC RA564.5 (eBook)
LC record available at https://lccn.loc.gov/2026007262
LC eBook record available at https://lccn.loc.gov/2026007263

CONTENTS

AT A GLANCE

- The mind and body are connected. It is important for people to take care of their physical well-being. This will support their mental health, too.
- Exercise helps strengthen muscles and bones. It also keeps the heart, brain, and lungs strong.
- Eating a balanced diet gives the body the energy and nutrients it needs to function.
- Teens need 8 to 10 hours of sleep every night. Sleep helps the brain focus and recharge.
- Drugs and alcohol can damage the body. They also worsen mental health.
- Stress is the body's response to physical or emotional danger. It is normal to feel stress sometimes. But too much stress can harm the body.

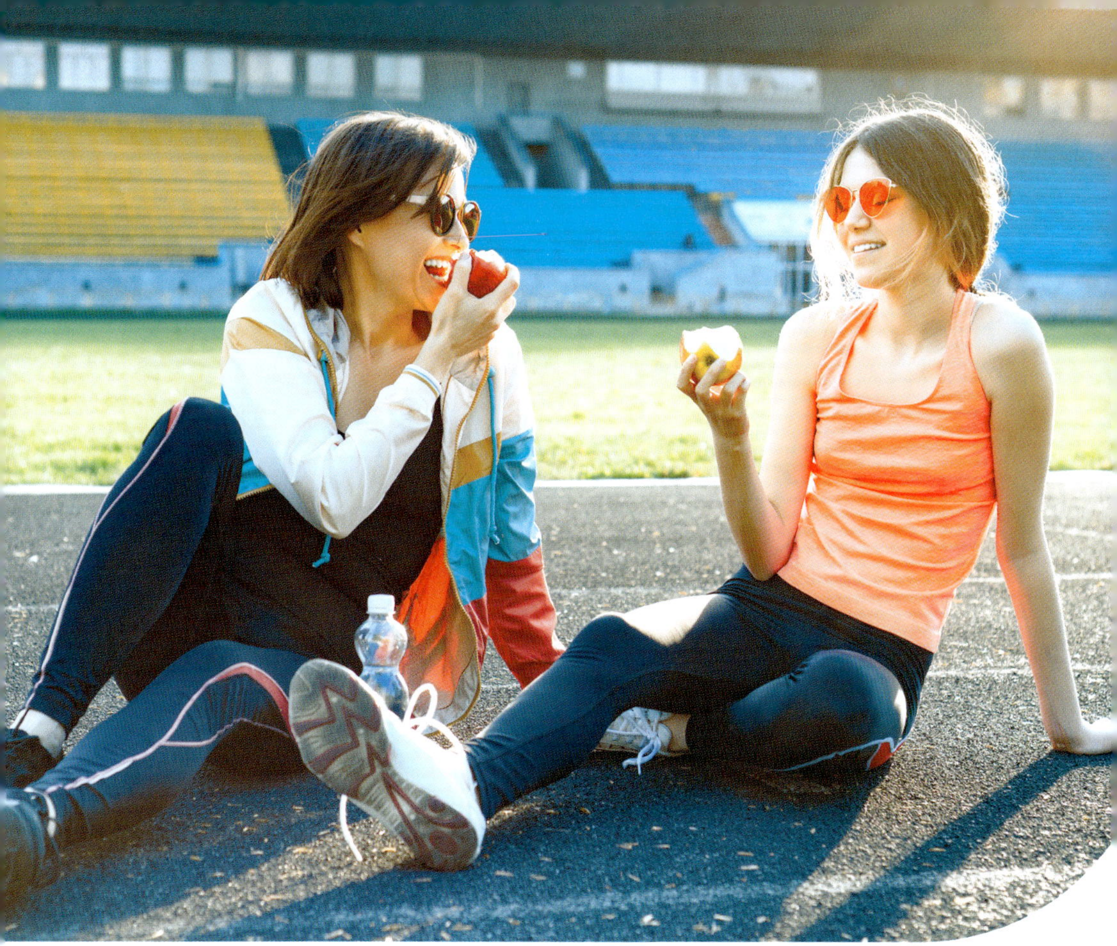

- People can practice gratitude and self-compassion to support their emotional well-being.
- Social well-being includes maintaining healthy relationships and connecting with others.
- People can work on their spiritual well-being by practicing mindfulness, identifying their values, and finding purpose in life.

VISITING THE DOCTOR

Tristan is an 18-year-old boy. He is at the doctor's office for his yearly visit. When he was a child, his mother would schedule these appointments. But this year, he started college. He made a goal to take care of his own health.

Tristan sits in the waiting room. He thinks about what a healthy life means to him. He tries to eat fruits and vegetables every day. In the evenings, he goes on walks.

During a yearly visit, doctors will perform a physical exam. They will ask patients questions about their physical and mental health. They may also talk about vaccines the patient needs.

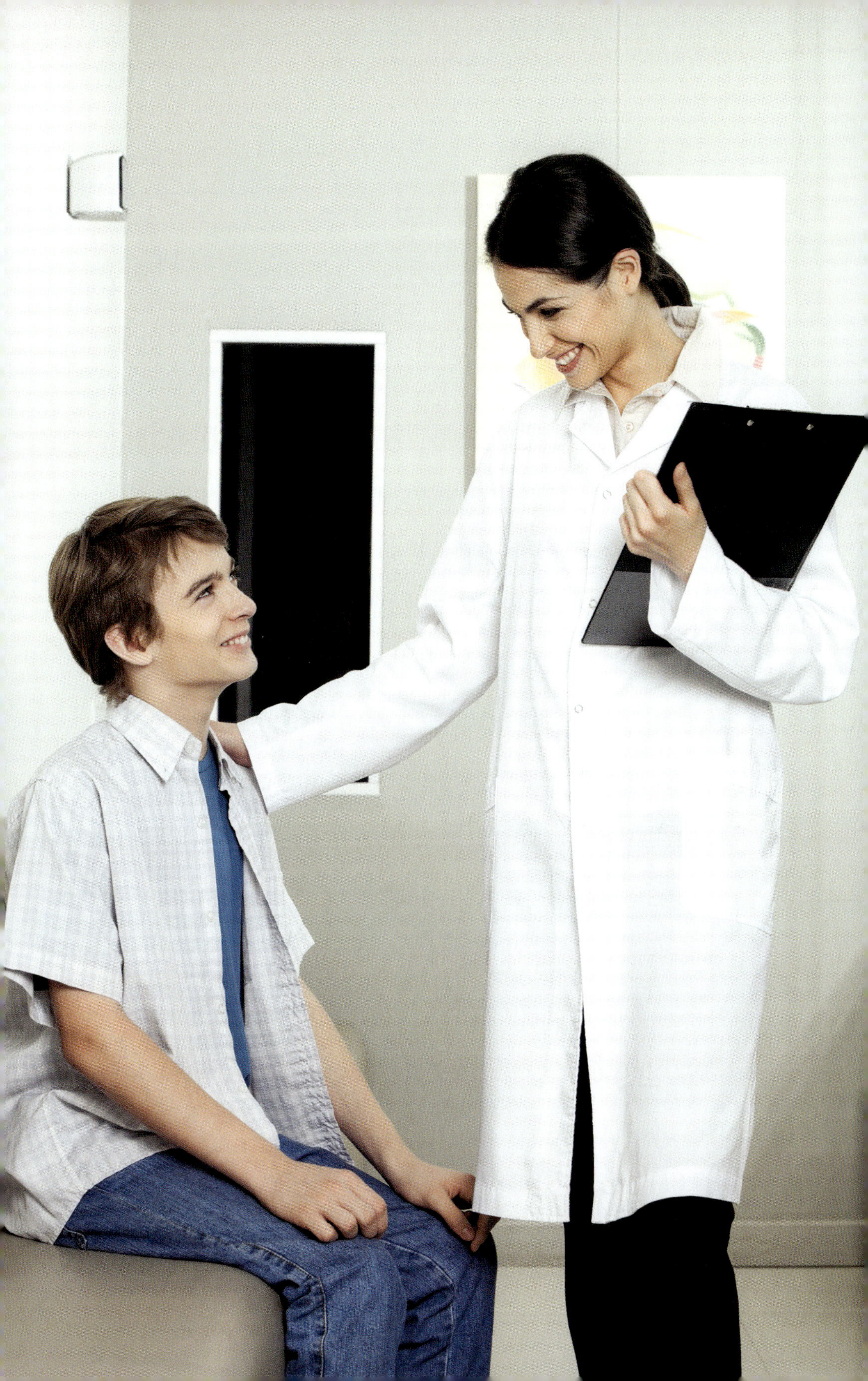

He **meditates** once in a while. He wonders if that is enough.

During the exam, Tristan's doctor listens to his heart and lungs. She asks Tristan about his health over the past year. When she is done, she asks if Tristan has questions.

Tristan tells her about his worries. "I try to take care of my body. I get sick sometimes. But how do I know if I'm healthy?"

The doctor tells Tristan that there are many ways to live a healthy life. And being healthy can mean something different for different people. "Being healthy does not mean being free from diseases," she says. "You are doing a great job of taking care of your body. You exercise, rest, and eat **nutritious** foods."

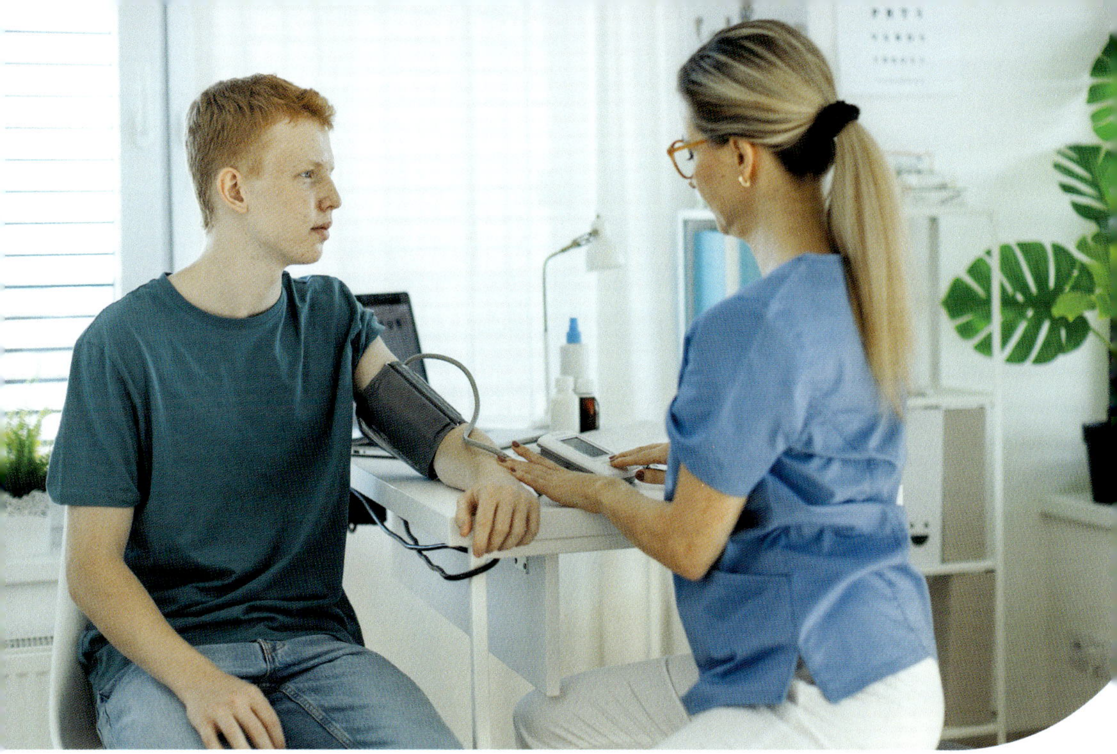

A physical exam includes checking a patient's blood pressure. Blood pressure measures how strongly the heart is bumping blood. High blood pressure can increase a person's risk of disease.

Tristan agrees. The doctor also asks Tristan how he manages stress. He says he talks to his friends and family about his feelings.

"It sounds like you're doing lots of good things!" the doctor says. "These are all ways to be healthy." Tristan leaves her office. He is proud of himself.

LIVING A HEALTHY LIFE

There are many things people can do to manage their health. Exercise, sleep, and nutrition support the body and brain. People can also build habits such as brushing their teeth twice a day. They can wear a seatbelt every time they are in a car. They can avoid tobacco.

Getting enough rest is important for all parts of a person's health. Sleep allows the body to recharge.

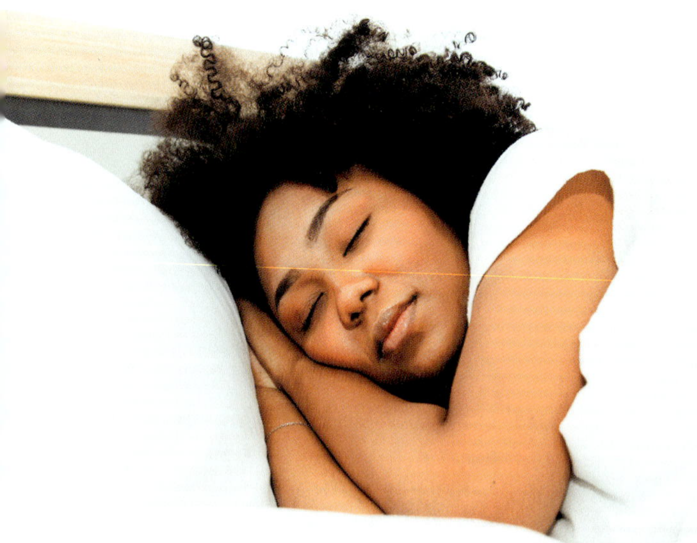

Mental health is important, too. This includes a person's social and emotional well-being. Valentina Ogaryan is a doctor specializing in cancer treatment. "To me, healthy refers to body, spirit, and mind," she said.[1]

The mind and body work together. When people take care of their bodies, their mental health also gets better. They are able to handle stress more easily. People can take care of their mental health by connecting with friends or family. They can also find enjoyable ways to relax.

Healthy activities look different for everyone. For example, people with different physical abilities may enjoy different types of exercise. Everyone can find ways to take care of their well-being.

EXERCISE AND NUTRITION

Two important ways to be healthy are exercising and eating nutritious foods. Exercise helps people strengthen their bodies. Nutrients help bodies function.

Some people think being healthy is only about being thin. But this is not true. The belief is also dangerous. It can make people harm themselves in order to lose weight. They may stop eating or exercise too much. People can be healthy in all kinds of bodies.

Playing team sports is one way to get regular exercise and have fun.

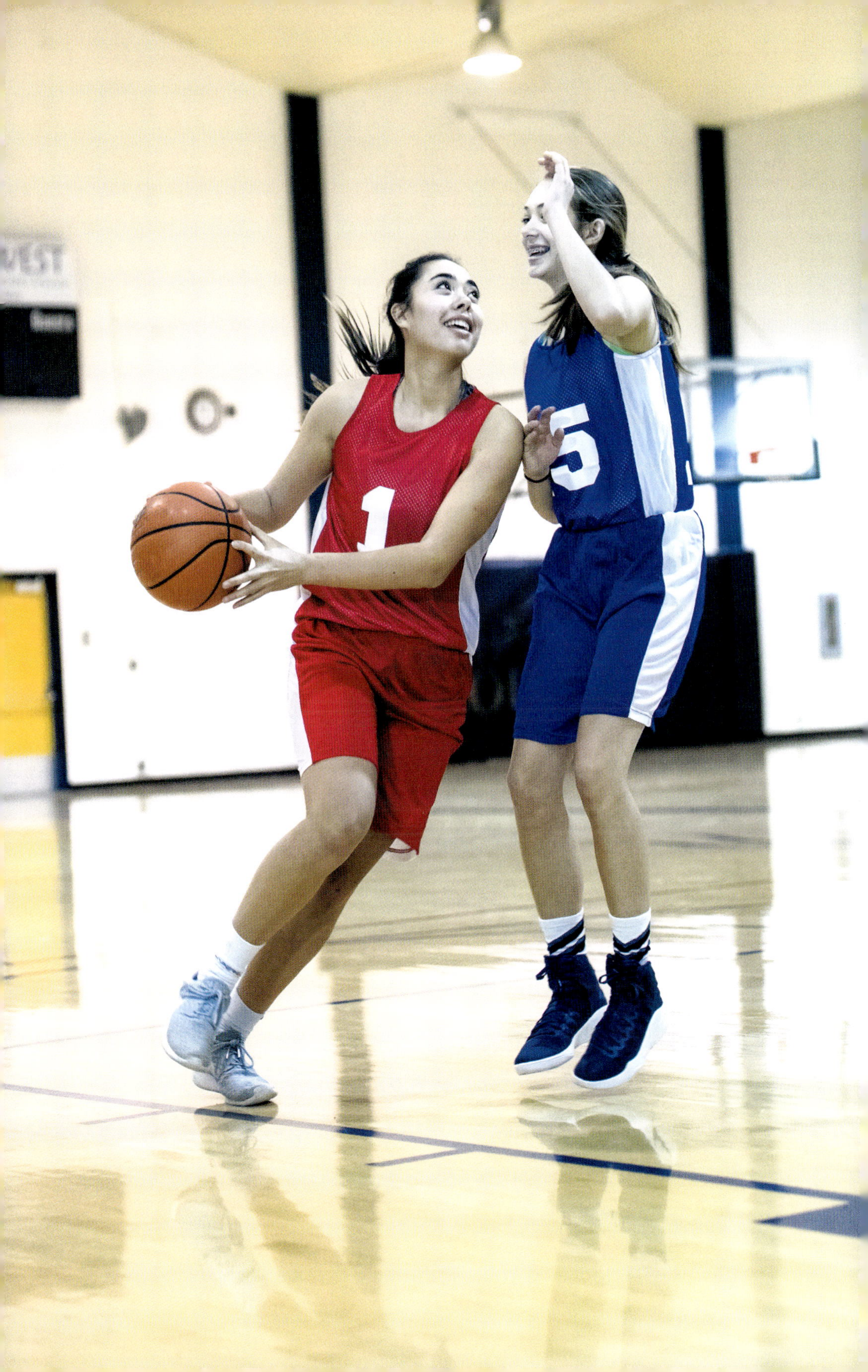

Exercising and eating a balanced diet may help people lose weight. But these habits are important for many more reasons, too. Rayven Nairn is a **dietician** with Johns Hopkins University. "It is time for us to shift away from weight-centric thinking and to [emphasize] body positivity, all-around health, and well-being," she says.[2]

IMPORTANCE OF EXERCISE

Exercise is good for every part of the body. It helps young people build strong bones and muscles. Exercising as a teenager builds healthy habits for life.

Exercise also keeps the heart in good shape. Being active helps the lungs send oxygen to the rest of the body. It helps blood flow to the brain. These are all important functions of the body.

Even mental health gets a boost from exercise. People who exercise can often handle stress better than those who do not. They are less likely to struggle with **mental illnesses**. Young people should

Body Image

Many young people are unhappy with their looks. This is called negative body image. Social media and societal messages can make people feel insecure. It's easy for people to compare themselves to others. But there are ways to improve body image. People can focus on what their bodies can do. They can think about what they need to be healthy. They can also make an effort to notice things they like about their looks. People who struggle with their body image can talk to a trusted adult or friend for help.

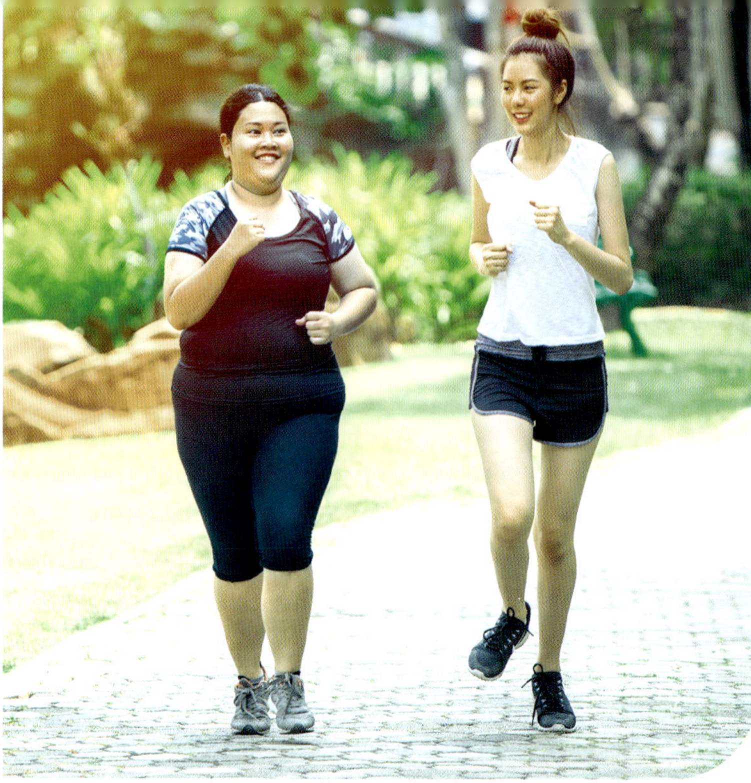

Running is a form of aerobic exercise. But it can be difficult for some people. Walking is another great way to get the heart pumping.

get at least an hour of physical activity every day.

FOUR TYPES OF EXERCISE

There are four types of exercise. They are aerobic, strengthening, stretching, and balance. Aerobic exercise is great for heart health. These activities make the heart pump blood faster. Swimming, biking, and dancing are examples of aerobic exercises.

Strength training is when the muscles push or pull against an object. This type of exercise builds muscle and bone. Some people lift weights or use weight-lifting machines. Others do strength training at home. Push-ups, sit-ups, and squats are strength exercises. It is important to do these exercises correctly. Doing them incorrectly can cause injuries.

Stretching helps the body stay flexible. When people stretch often, they are less likely to hurt their muscles. Stretching before and after other types of exercise helps reduce the risk of injury.

Balance helps with **coordination**. Without it, people can fall over and get hurt more easily. One way to practice balance is standing on one foot. Another is walking from toe to heel in a straight line.

The best types of exercise for a person are the ones that they enjoy and can do every day. When people have fun, they are motivated to exercise. The more they exercise, the more it becomes a habit and helps their bodies. People can also find the types of movement that work best for their bodies. People with physical disabilities might have different exercise strategies than those without disabilities.

Variety is important, too. Different exercises help different parts of the body. A varied exercise plan includes aerobic, strength, stretching, and balance activities every week.

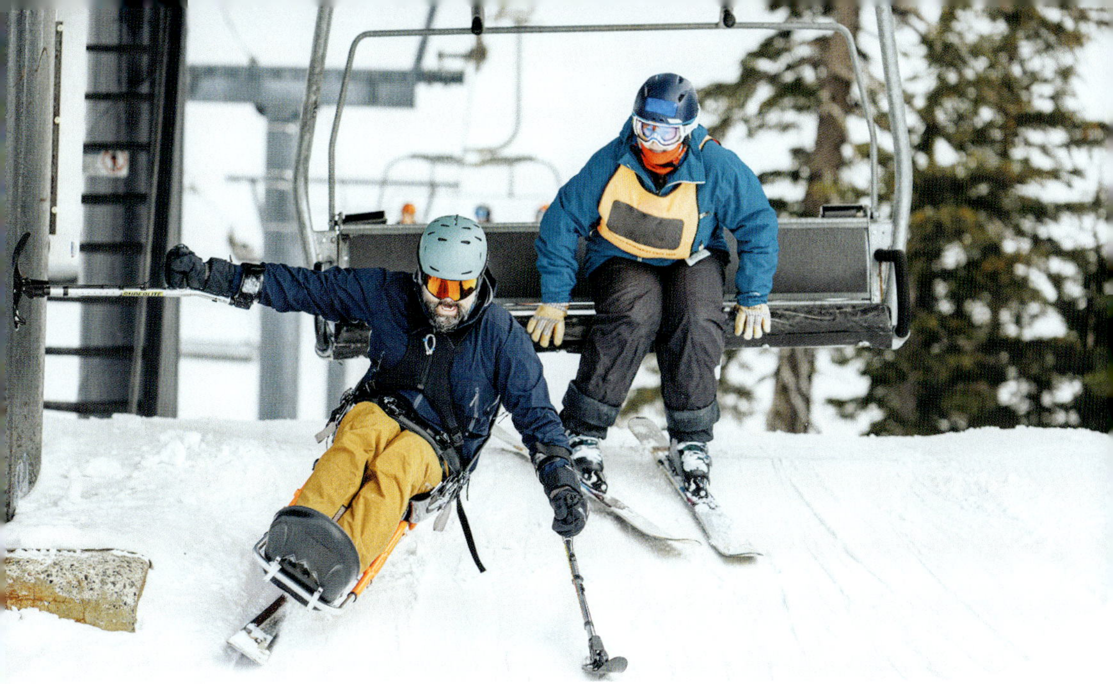

Adaptive sports equipment can help people with disabilities participate in a variety of activities.

Many people work out at a gym or rec center. This can make exercise easier, but it is not necessary. Many exercises don't need special equipment. Dancing, running, and jumping jacks are a few examples.

NUTRITION

Some people think healthy eating means following fad diets. These are **restrictive** eating plans. They may tell people to eat

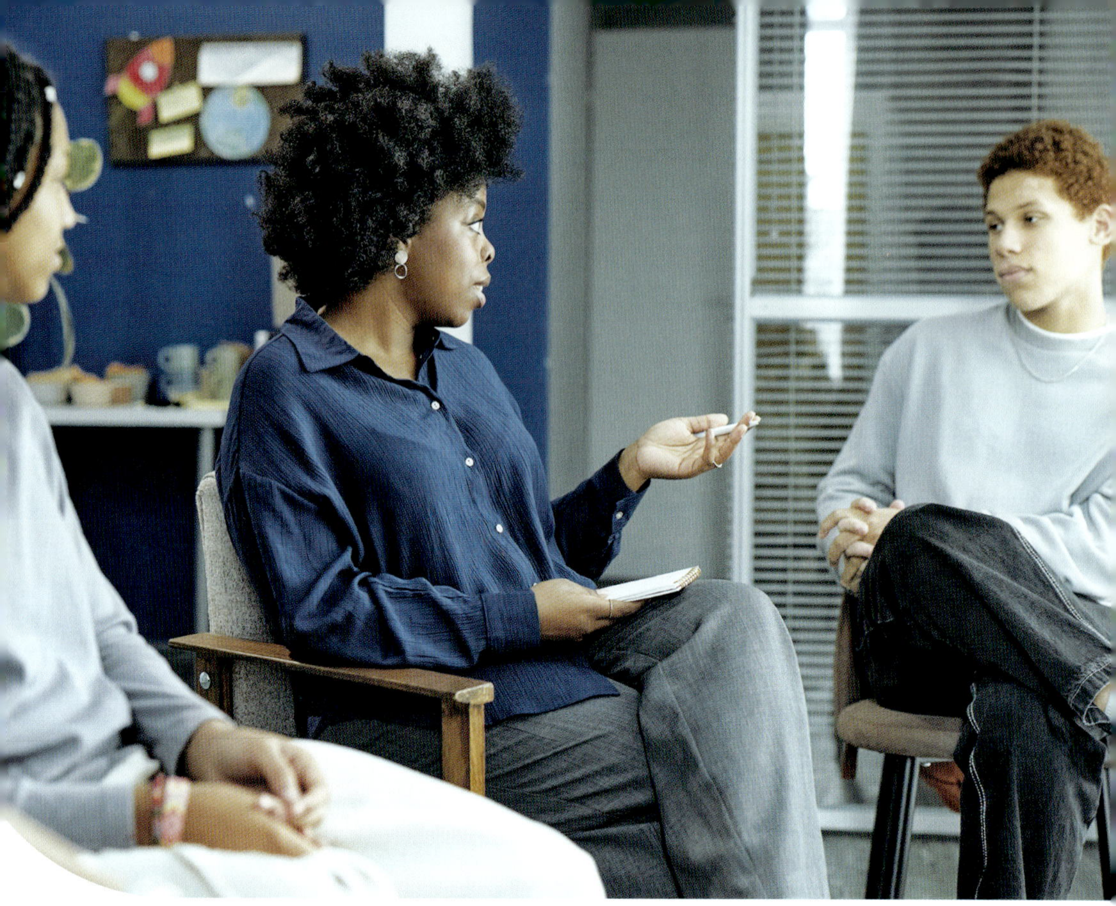

Eating disorders are dangerous illnesses that affect a person's eating habits and thoughts about food and appearance. Doctors and therapists can help people struggling with eating disorders.

only certain types of food. Or they may tell people to eat only small amounts of food.

The guidelines are difficult to follow. They may leave people feeling hungry and unsatisfied. They can also lead to feelings of failure if a person cannot continue the diet.

Following fad diets can be harmful to people's physical and mental health.

Instead, people can focus on eating a balanced diet. Venus Kalami is a dietician who works with young people. "One of the main things I advocate for is minimizing unnecessary restriction and loosening it up so we can get some flexibility, freedom, and variety back in our lives," she says.[3]

FIVE FOOD GROUPS

There are five main groups of foods. These are fruits, vegetables, grains, proteins, and dairy. Each one provides important nutrients for the body. People should aim to eat a balance of these five types of foods.

Fruits and vegetables have vitamins, minerals, and fiber. Vitamins and minerals help the body function. They also help people avoid illnesses. Fiber helps the body's **digestive** system.

Grains have fiber, vitamins, and minerals, too. They provide people with energy. Whole grains such as oatmeal, brown rice, and wheat bread have the most nutrients. Refined grains such as white bread have fewer nutrients. People should focus on eating mostly whole grains.

The body uses protein to build bone, muscle, and blood. Fish, beans, and lean meat such as chicken all have protein. Dairy products, such as milk and cheese, also keep bones strong. Soy products can provide nutrients to people who can't eat dairy. Soy drinks or yogurts with calcium are especially nutritious.

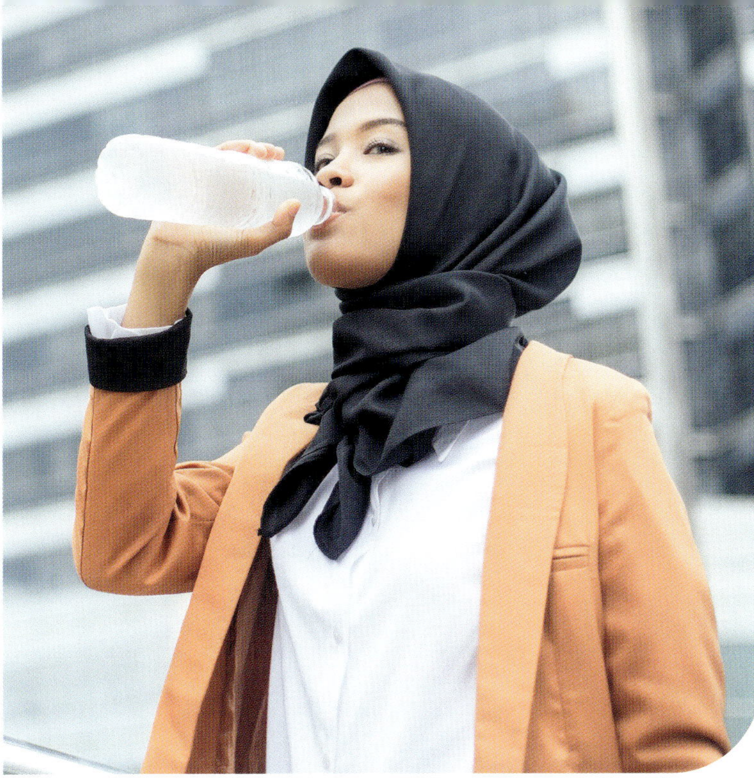

It is important to drink plenty of water throughout the day. Drinks such as soda, juice, and energy drinks can add a lot of sugar to a person's diet.

A balanced diet will look different for everyone. Some people enjoy certain foods more than others. Some people have allergies or other dietary restrictions that limit their access to certain food groups. But everyone should try to add variety to their diets. Each of the five food groups has benefits.

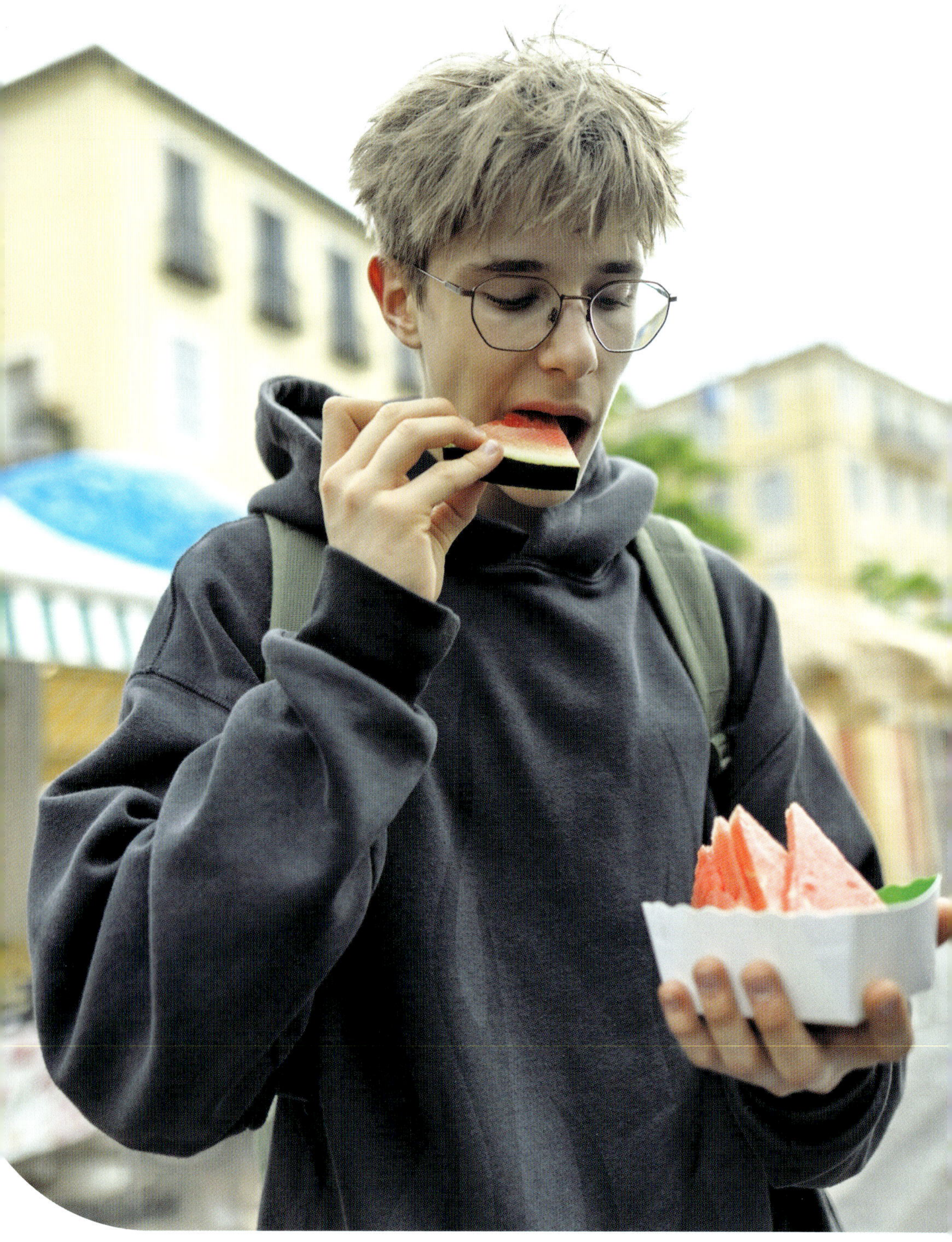

Eating fruits and vegetables as snacks is one way to avoid processed foods with lots of salt and sugar.

PROCESSED FOODS

Processed foods are foods that have been changed in some way. Some foods are more processed than others. Canned beans are one example of a processed food. Pop-Tarts are another.

Ultra-processed foods often have a lot of salt and sugar. Eating too much sugar and salt is harmful. Brent M. Egan is a doctor who specializes in internal organs and heart health. "A general principle is if you can eat foods that are less processed—fruits, vegetables, whole grains, most meat—it is better for you," he says.[4] Processed foods can be part of a healthy diet in limited amounts. But balance is key.

CHAPTER TWO

BRAIN HEALTH

The brain needs care just like the rest of the body. The brain controls everything a person does during the day. It also helps them rest and recharge at night.

A healthy brain is important for the body and mind. It is important to protect the brain from physical injury. For example, people can wear helmets when riding bikes. Good daily habits can also help protect the brain.

An athlete can avoid injuring their brain by wearing a helmet. Helmets are especially important in sports where players might hit their heads.

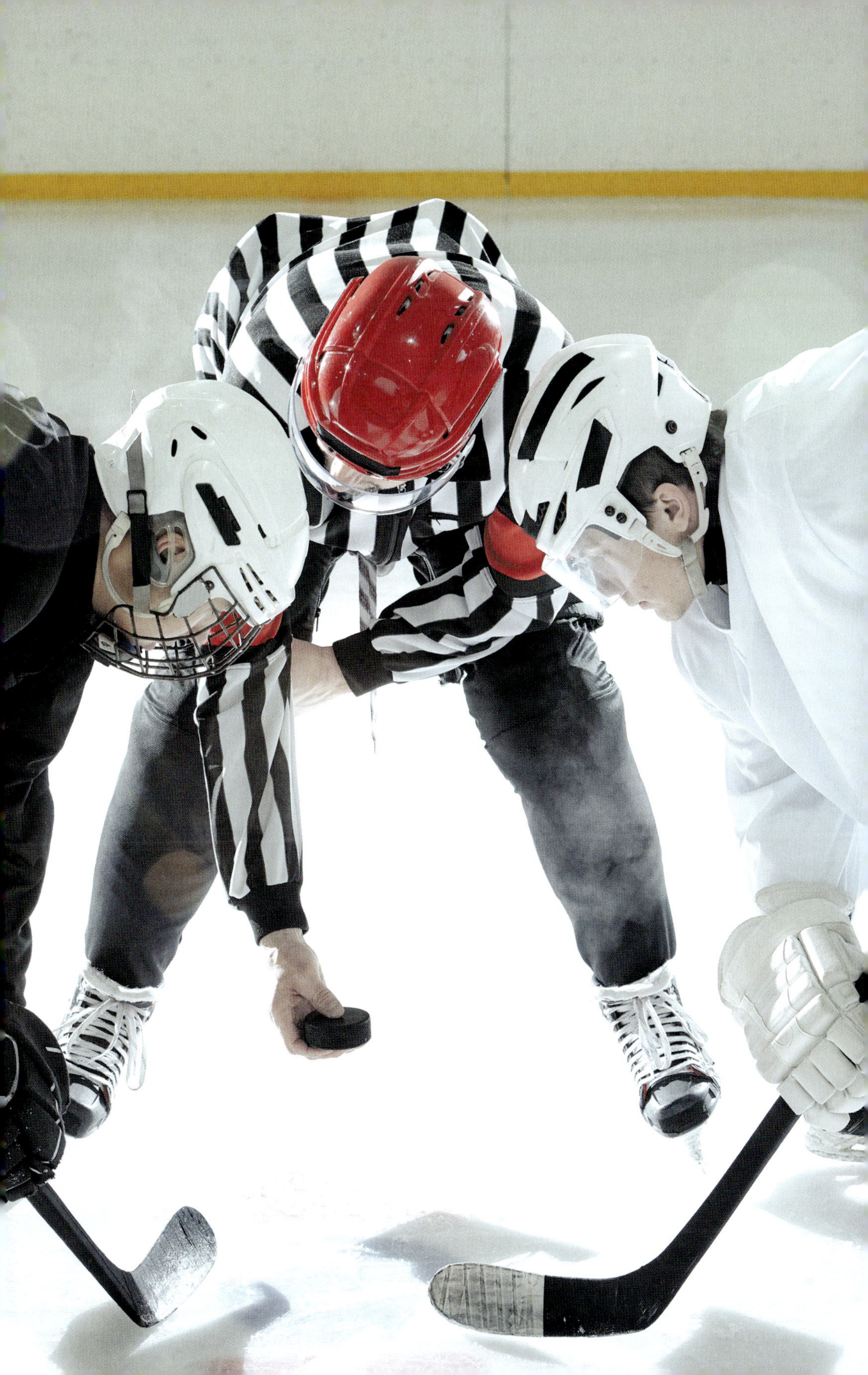

Exercise, nutrition, sleep, and other choices all affect brain health.

ALCOHOL AND DRUGS

The US government makes laws that limit people's access to alcohol and drugs, including tobacco. There are good reasons for these laws. Drugs and alcohol affect how the brain works. They make

The Dangers of E-Cigarettes

E-cigarettes are also called vapes. They are a newer invention than cigarettes. Some people assume they are safer for that reason. This is not true. Vapes are just as addictive as cigarettes. Most teens who start vaping want to quit. It can be hard, but it is never too late. People who are struggling to quit using vapes can talk to a parent, teacher, or another trusted adult for help.

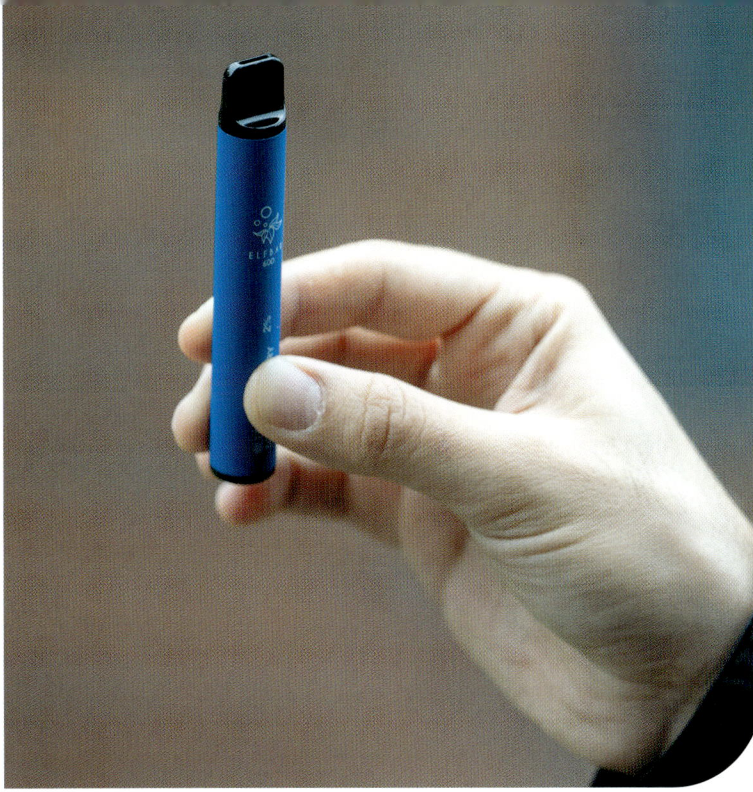

E-cigarettes, or vapes, may not look harmful. But they are. They are also addictive. It can be difficult for a person to quit using them after they start.

it harder to think clearly and make good decisions. Drugs and alcohol can affect the development of young people's brains. This causes long-term damage. Drugs and alcohol can also damage the heart, liver, and other organs.

People may become addicted to drugs or alcohol. Over time, their bodies rely on the substance more and more. They may feel sick if they don't take it every day. They may need help from a doctor to quit. People might also take more of a substance or substances than the body can handle. This is called an overdose. Overdosing causes serious problems. It can even lead to death.

In the United States, it is illegal for people under 21 years old to drink alcohol, use tobacco products, or consume marijuana. Many other drugs are illegal for everyone. People may feel pressured to use illegal substances. But it is important to make safe, healthy choices instead.

SLEEP

When people sleep, the brain gets important work done. It stores what a person learned during the day in their memory. It also prepares them to focus the next day.

The amount of sleep people need often changes as they get older. Young people

One sign that a person is getting enough sleep is that they wake up feeling refreshed.

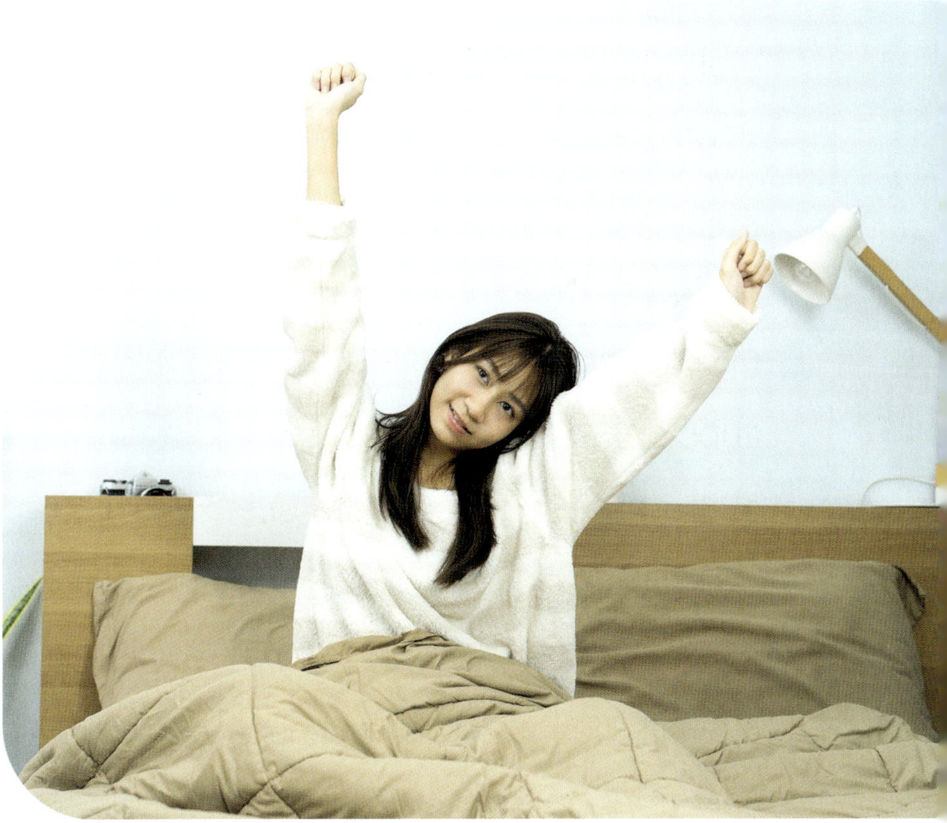

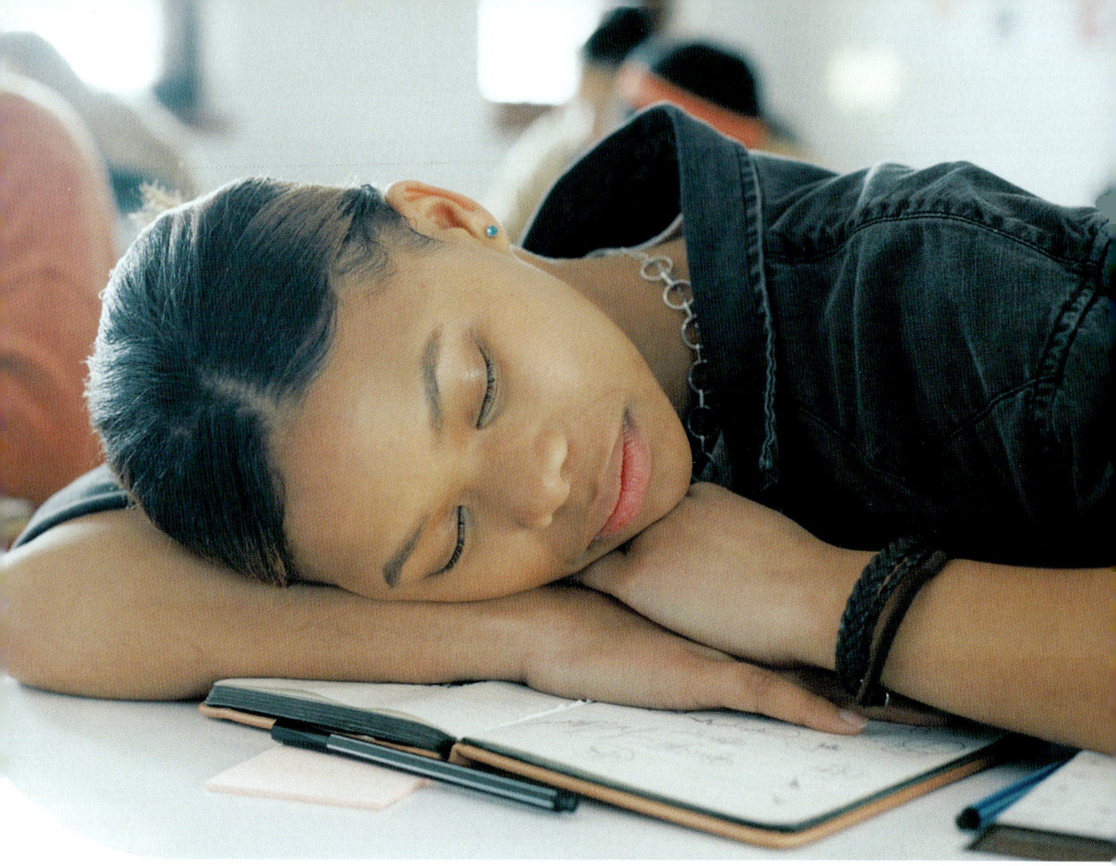

Some people get tired in the middle of the school day. Eating a healthy snack, getting some fresh air, and stretching the body are ways to feel more alert.

generally need more sleep than adults. Teenagers should aim for 8 to 10 hours of sleep each night. The exact number is different for everyone. People can pay attention to what works for their bodies.

Most people know getting enough sleep is important. But some people struggle to fall asleep. A sleep routine may help. Going to sleep and waking up at the same time every day helps many people get better sleep.

It's also important to avoid certain things before bedtime. The bright light of screens can keep the brain awake. People should put their digital devices in another room when it's time to sleep. Caffeine can also make it hard to fall asleep. Caffeine stays in the blood for up to 12 hours. Drinking it too close to bedtime can make sleeping difficult. People should avoid consuming caffeine in the afternoon and evening.

Some people have insomnia. This is when a person struggles to sleep at least three times a week. They may wake up a lot at night. They may feel tired during the day, too. People who struggle with insomnia should see a doctor. Medical professionals can help find a cause and treat it.

BRAIN FITNESS

Like the body, the brain needs exercise. People should plan activities that challenge their brain every day. These will help strengthen the skills they need for school, work, and daily life.

Nurse practitioner Kelsey Kidd says, "There are many things that you can do to keep your brain in shape, such as doing crossword puzzles or sudoku, reading, playing cards or putting together a jigsaw puzzle."[5] Learning a language is another challenge for the brain. Young people pick up new languages more quickly than adults.

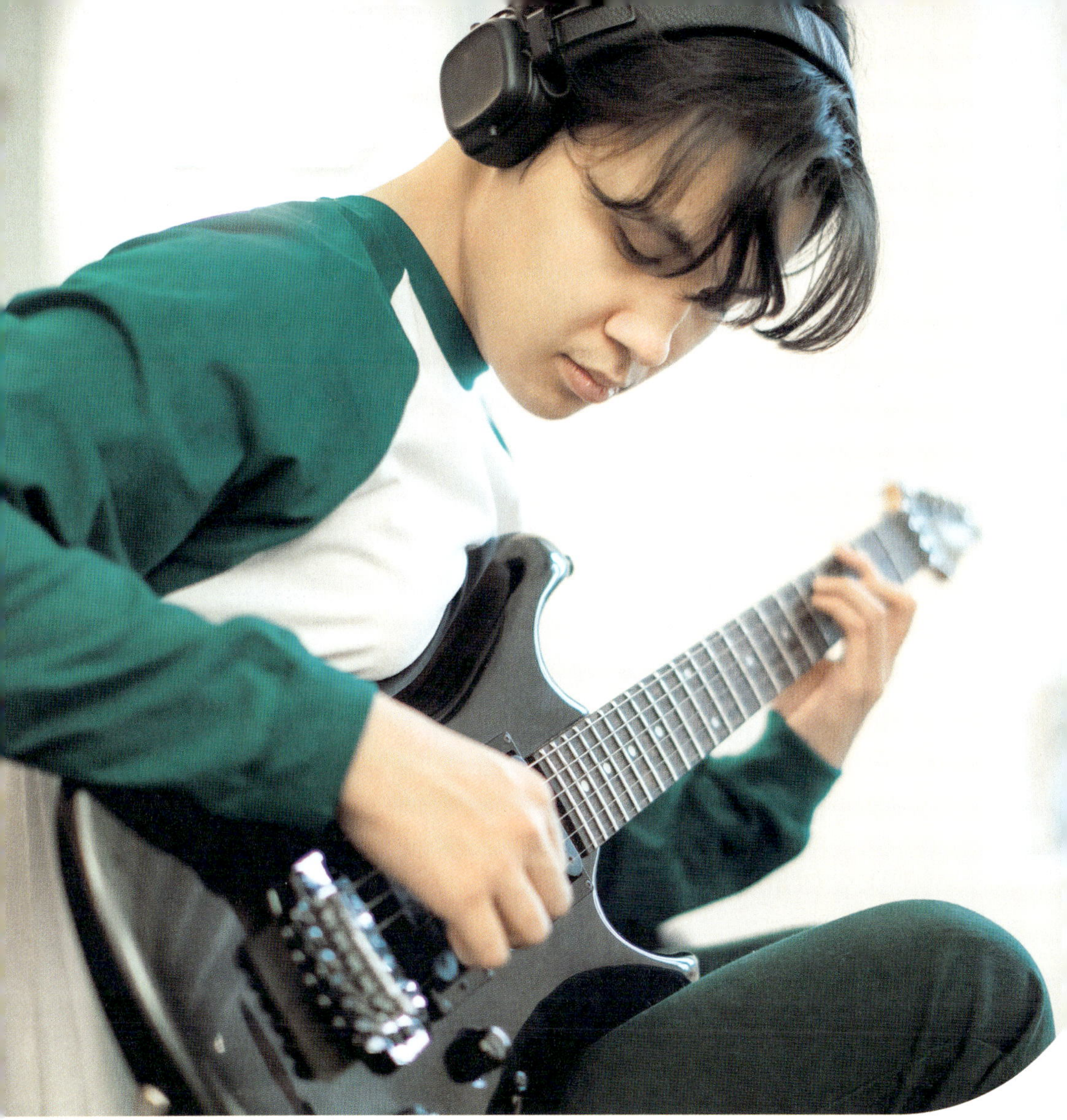

Practicing an instrument is one way to keep a sharp brain. It can also reduce stress and improve mental health.

Their brains are open to learning different grammar skills. Studying a new language can help keep the brain sharp.

CHAPTER THREE

MENTAL HEALTH

Mental health affects how people think and feel. It also affects how people handle their emotions. Some people struggle with mental illnesses such as depression or anxiety. It is important for all people to take care of their mental health.

Daily habits can support mental well-being. They can also prevent mental health emergencies. People can learn

Writing in a journal helps some people process their emotions. This can boost their mental health.

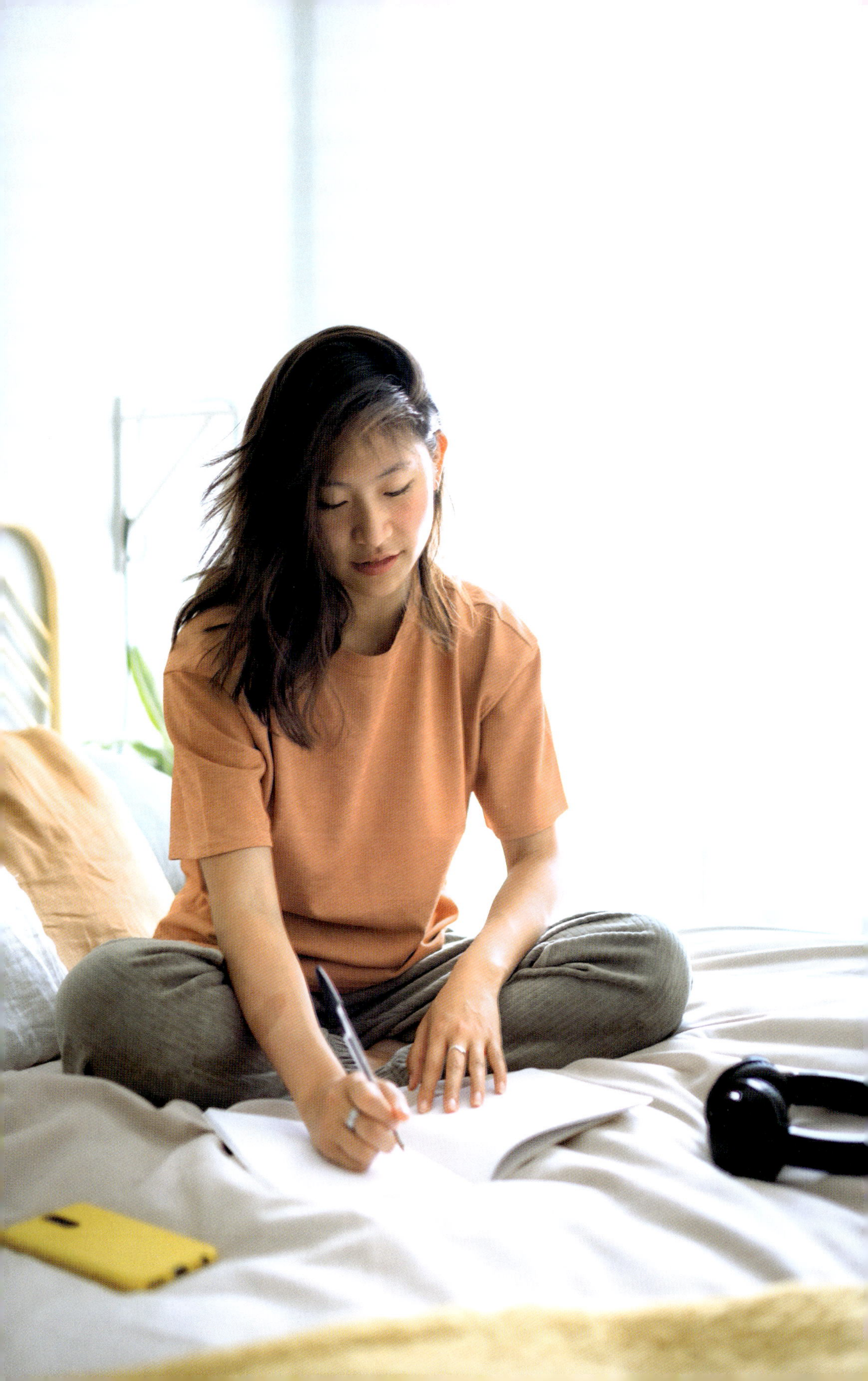

tools for when they are struggling with their mental health.

MANAGING STRESS

Stress is how the body responds to danger. Sometimes physical danger causes stress. But many other situations cause stress, too. These may include school deadlines

Spending time outside can help people reduce their stress.

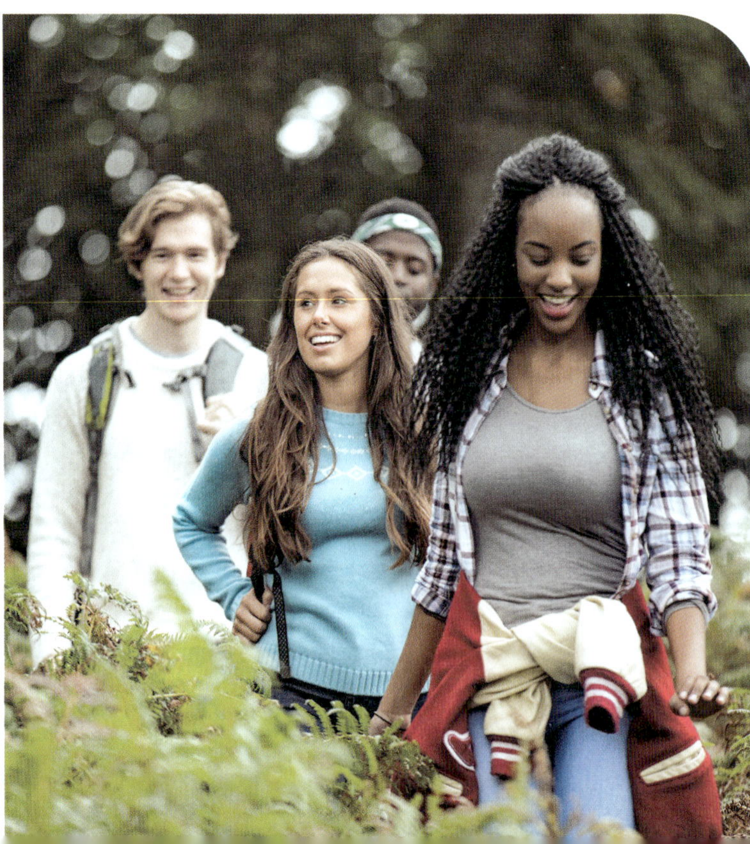

and social conflicts. In stressful situations, the body goes into alert mode. The heart beats faster and muscles tense up. The body releases a chemical called adrenaline. Adrenaline gives people energy to face danger.

It's normal to feel stress sometimes. But constant stress takes a toll. Too much stress can give people headaches, stomachaches, and muscle tension. It can even cause heart problems over time.

Everyone has different stressors in life. Some mental illnesses also make stress more difficult to manage. There are steps people can take to lower their stress. But if a person is struggling to manage their stress on their own, they should ask a trusted adult for help.

5-4-3-2-1 GROUNDING

Start by taking long, slow breaths. Then notice:

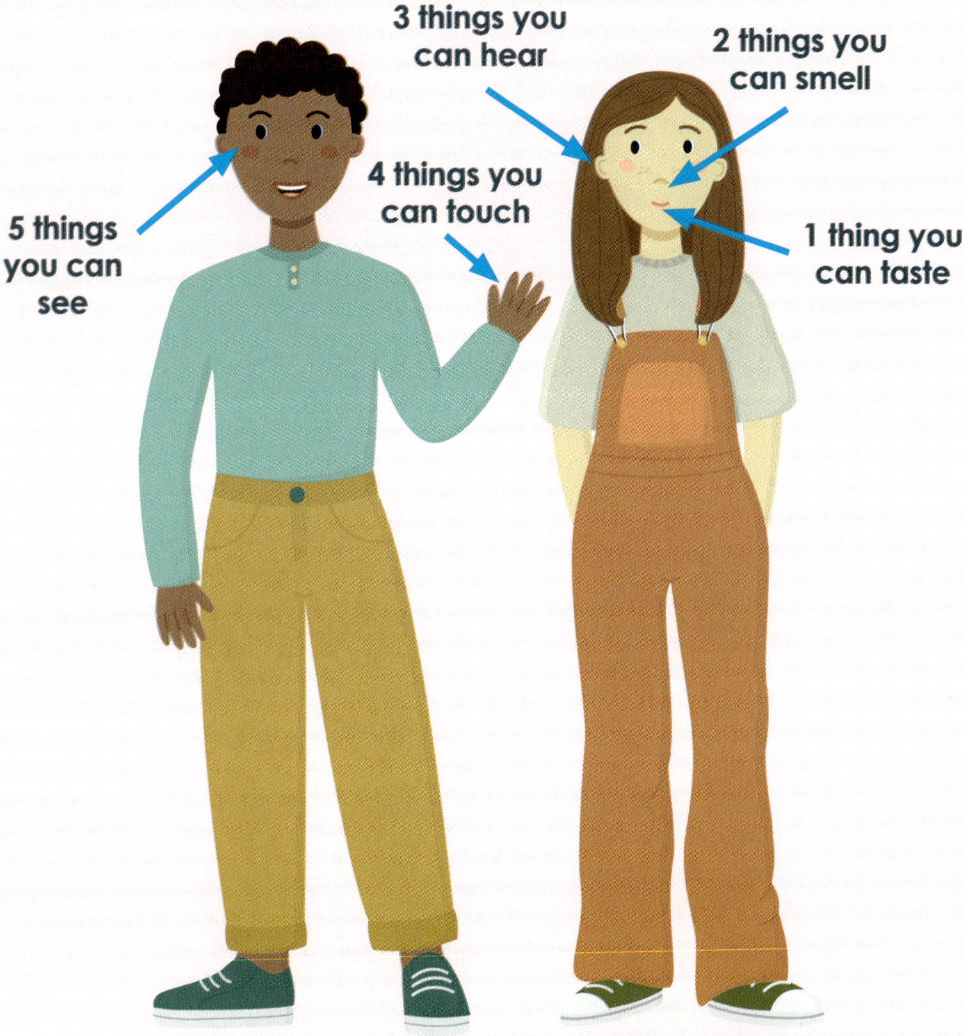
3 things you can hear
2 things you can smell
4 things you can touch
5 things you can see
1 thing you can taste

Sometimes people feel a huge amount of stress or anxiety. They can use grounding exercises to help calm down. These are tools to help a person connect with their body and slow their mind. One grounding exercise helps people connect to their five senses.

Taking deep breaths is one stress reliever. It helps with physical symptoms, including a racing heart. Box breathing is a popular technique. First, a person breathes in slowly while counting to four. Then they hold their breath for four counts. Next, they breathe out for four counts. Finally, they hold their breath again for four counts. They repeat this cycle until their body calms down.

People can also reduce stress by learning to manage their time. Deadlines can be a big stressor. Students can reduce their stress by breaking big projects into small steps. When a test is coming up, they can take time to study for a little while every day. They can also ask the teacher questions about any confusing topics.

These steps will help keep stress at manageable levels.

Sometimes people turn to unhealthy habits when they are stressed. They may drink alcohol, take drugs, or hurt themselves. They may also use social media or video games to avoid their stress.

Hope Squad

Hope Squad is a volunteer program with a mission to save lives. Students learn about the warning signs of a mental health crisis. They connect classmates who are struggling with adults who can help. Maddie is a Hope Squad volunteer. She says, "It's hard to have these conversations but, as we work together, we learn how to take care of ourselves while taking care of other people."

Quoted in Sara Weber, "What One Utah Student Learned in Hope Squad Helped Her Save a Friend's Life," Hope Squad, *May 7, 2024. www.hopesquad.com.*

These all make stress worse over time. People who are struggling to manage stress should talk to a trusted adult for help.

GRATITUDE

Gratitude means noticing and appreciating the good parts of life. People can practice paying attention to the little things that make them happy. When people focus on what they are thankful for, their mental health can get better. Gratitude can also make people better prepared to deal with stress.

Life can be tough. Being grateful doesn't mean ignoring pain or sadness. Instead, it reminds people why they keep going. It helps them build **resilience**.

Some people like to list a few things they're grateful for every day. They might write these thoughts in a gratitude journal. This habit can have positive effects on well-being.

SELF-COMPASSION

Many people are too hard on themselves. When they make mistakes, they think unkind things. Everyone has an inner critic. But when that voice is too loud, it can make people ashamed of who they are.

Self-compassion is when people treat themselves kindly. People might practice treating themselves like a friend. Most people would not yell at a friend when they make a mistake. They would cheer their friend up and help them try again. When people are kind to themselves, they handle stress better.

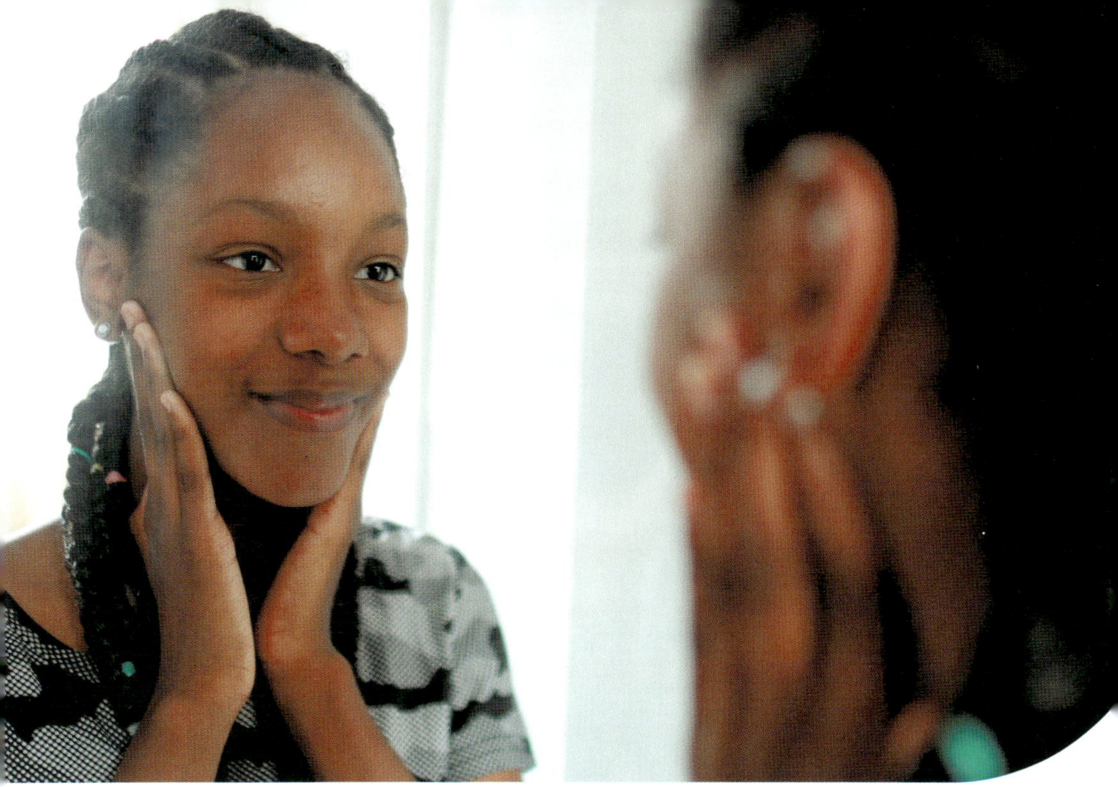

Affirmations are positive statements people say to themselves every day. Saying affirmations can help with self-compassion.

Kristin Neff studies and teaches about self-compassion. She says,

> *Whenever I notice something about myself I don't like, I silently repeat the following phrases: This is a moment of suffering. Suffering is part of life. May I be kind to myself at this moment. May I give myself the compassion I need.*[6]

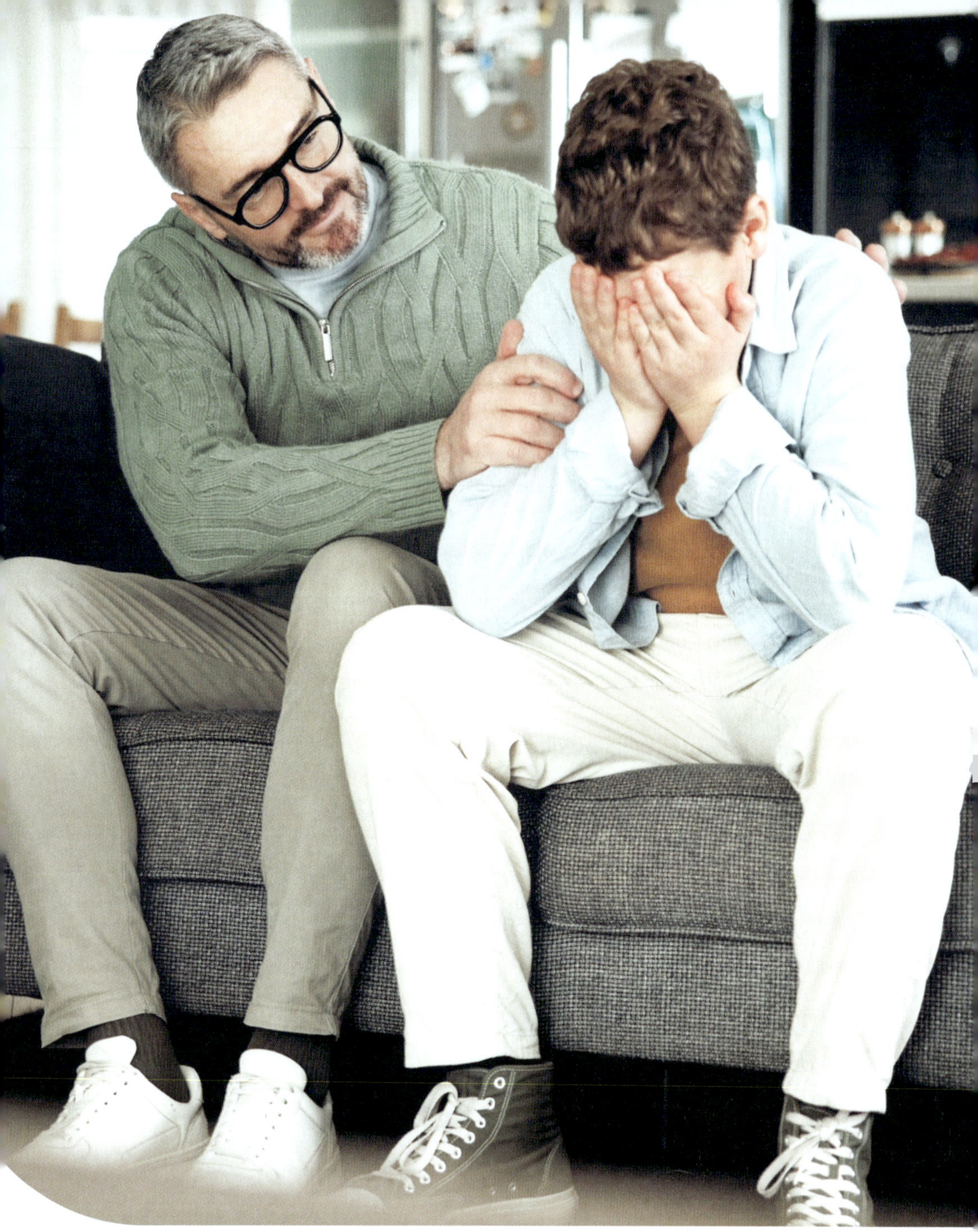

Thinking about hurting oneself or others are serious signs of a mental health crisis. A person with these feelings should talk to a trusted adult right away.

SIGNS OF A MENTAL HEALTH CRISIS

Some issues are too big to solve alone. Everyone feels sad or worried sometimes. But it's not normal to feel upset most of the time. That can be a sign of mental illness.

People should learn to notice other signs of mental illness. These include avoiding friends and family, not feeling hungry anymore, feeling hopeless, and struggling to focus. When these signs affect a person's day-to-day life, the person needs help. A doctor or therapist can help people struggling with their mental health. People can learn skills to help manage their emotions. Or a doctor might prescribe medication to help manage their symptoms.

CHAPTER FOUR

SOCIAL AND SPIRITUAL WELL-BEING

Relationships are important for living a long and happy life. They are a part of social well-being. Author Casper ter Kuile says, "Being truly connected isn't a luxury. It's a lifesaver."[7] Spending time with friends, family, or other loved ones keeps people healthy.

Human brains need close relationships. Relationships are a basic need similar to food and water. Quality is more important

It is important for young people to have healthy relationships. These can include romantic relationships and relationships with friends and family.

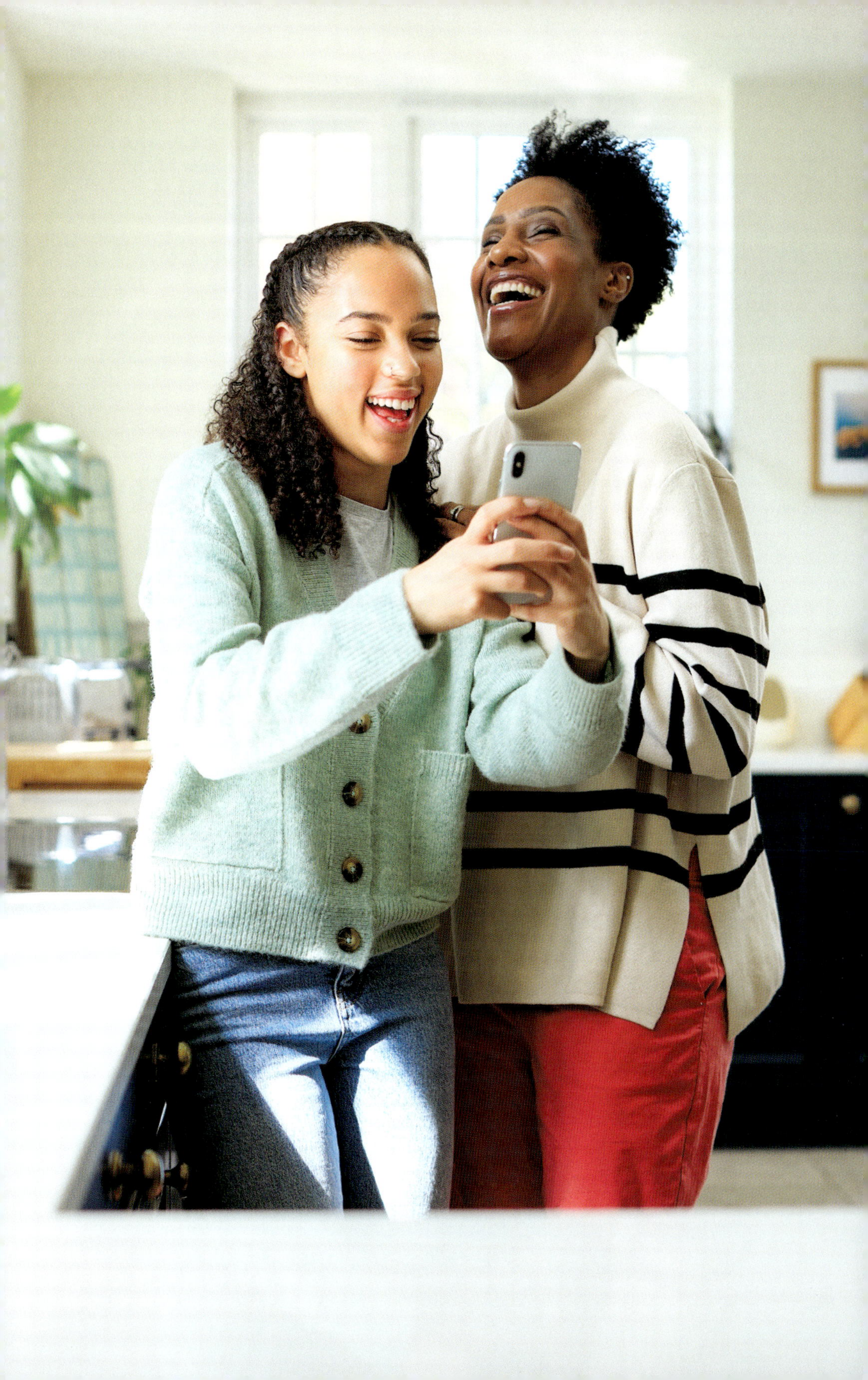

than quantity. That means it's better to have a few close friends than to be around many casual friends.

HOW TO CONNECT WITH OTHERS

Making friends is not always easy. Some people have conditions such as autism or social anxiety disorders that affect social skills. Others may feel anxious around people they don't know.

It can help to start small. People can try to smile or say hello to someone new every day. As people open up, they may feel more comfortable around others. They may even connect with someone they didn't expect.

People can also build community by joining hobby groups. These are groups of people who have similar interests.

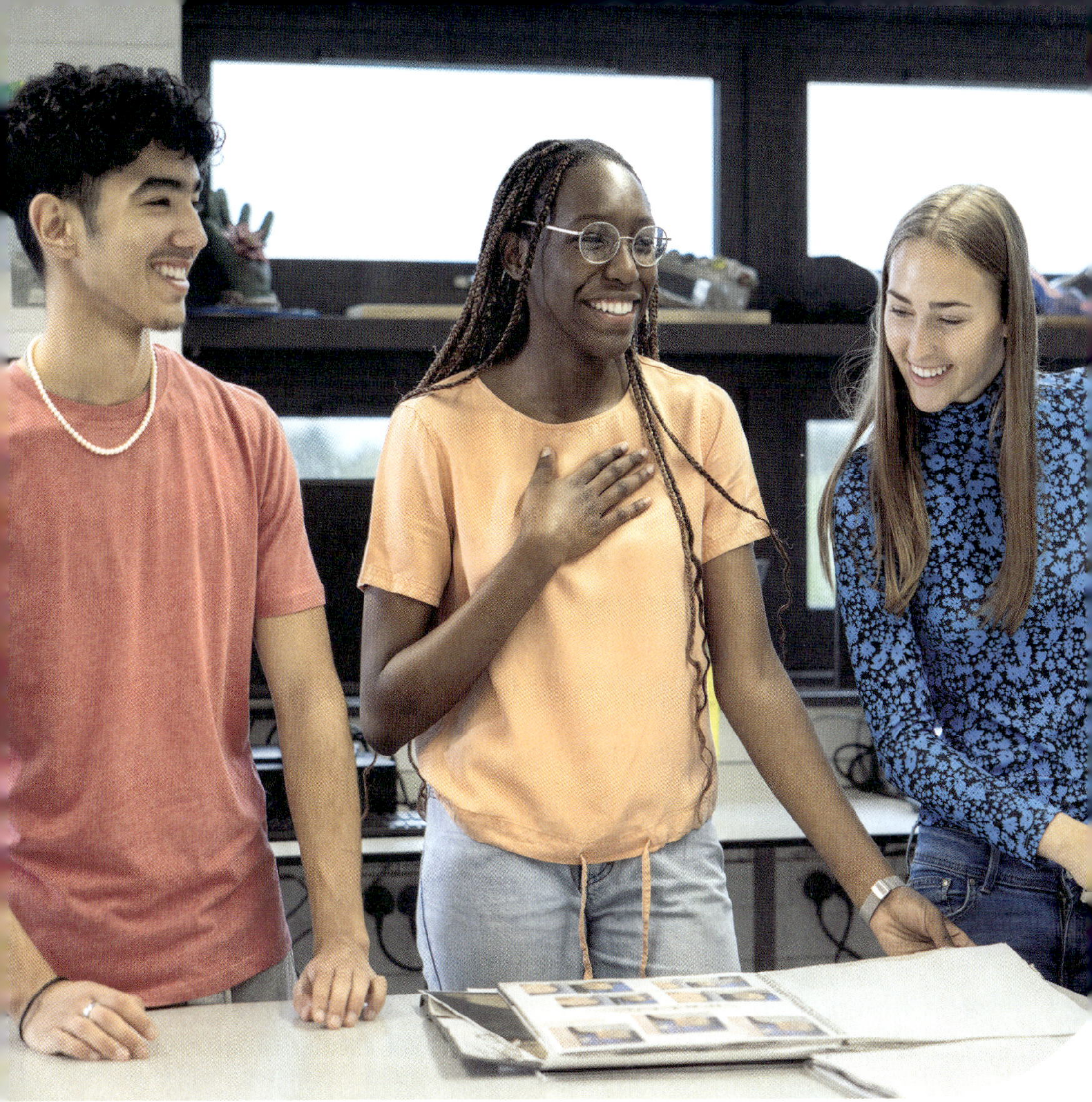

School clubs can be great places to meet new people with similar interests.

They might all like to draw or play basketball. These groups can be a good place to meet friends. Members know they have something in common.

Volunteering is a good way to give back to a community. Volunteering often reduces stress. Volunteers feel connected to the people around them. It helps people to choose a cause they are passionate about. People who love animals might volunteer at a pet shelter. People who love books could help at the library.

SPIRITUALITY

Many people think spirituality is the same thing as religion. Spirituality can include religion. But it doesn't have to. It's about finding purpose and connection. It helps people feel like they belong to something bigger than themselves.

Mindfulness can help people explore spirituality. When people are mindful, they

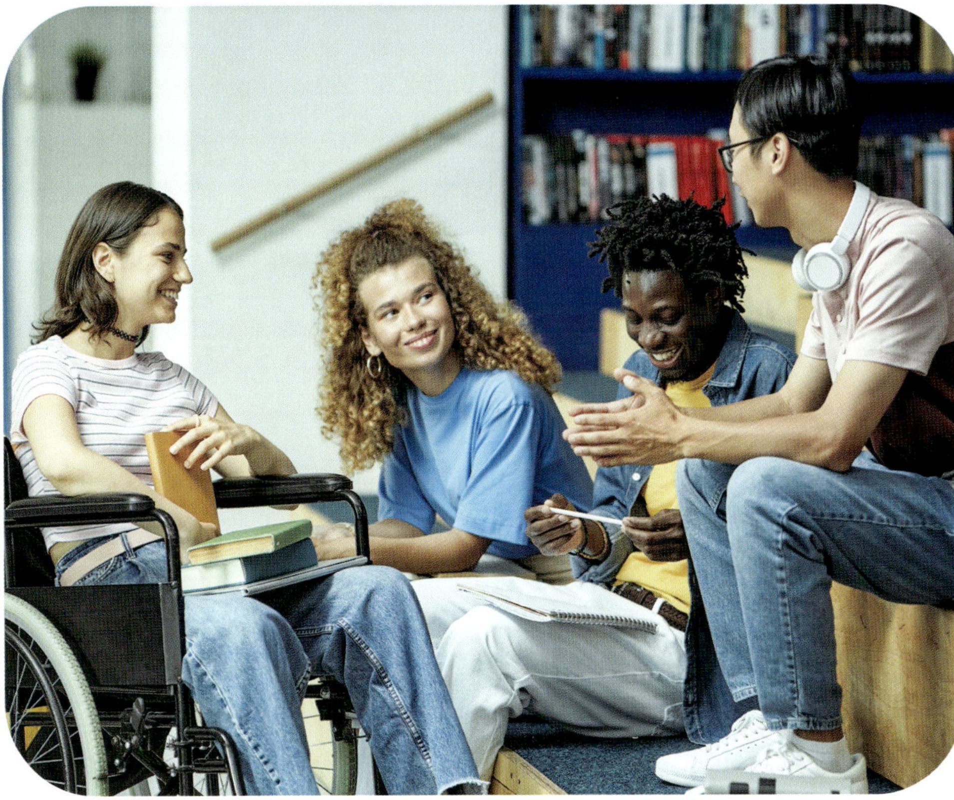

Talking to people with different religions, philosophies, and belief systems can help people learn about different ways to practice spirituality.

pay attention to the present. They might meditate. Or they may go on a quiet walk and notice how their bodies feel. They look around. They listen. They let go of their worries.

Loving-kindness meditation is one way to practice mindfulness. It teaches people

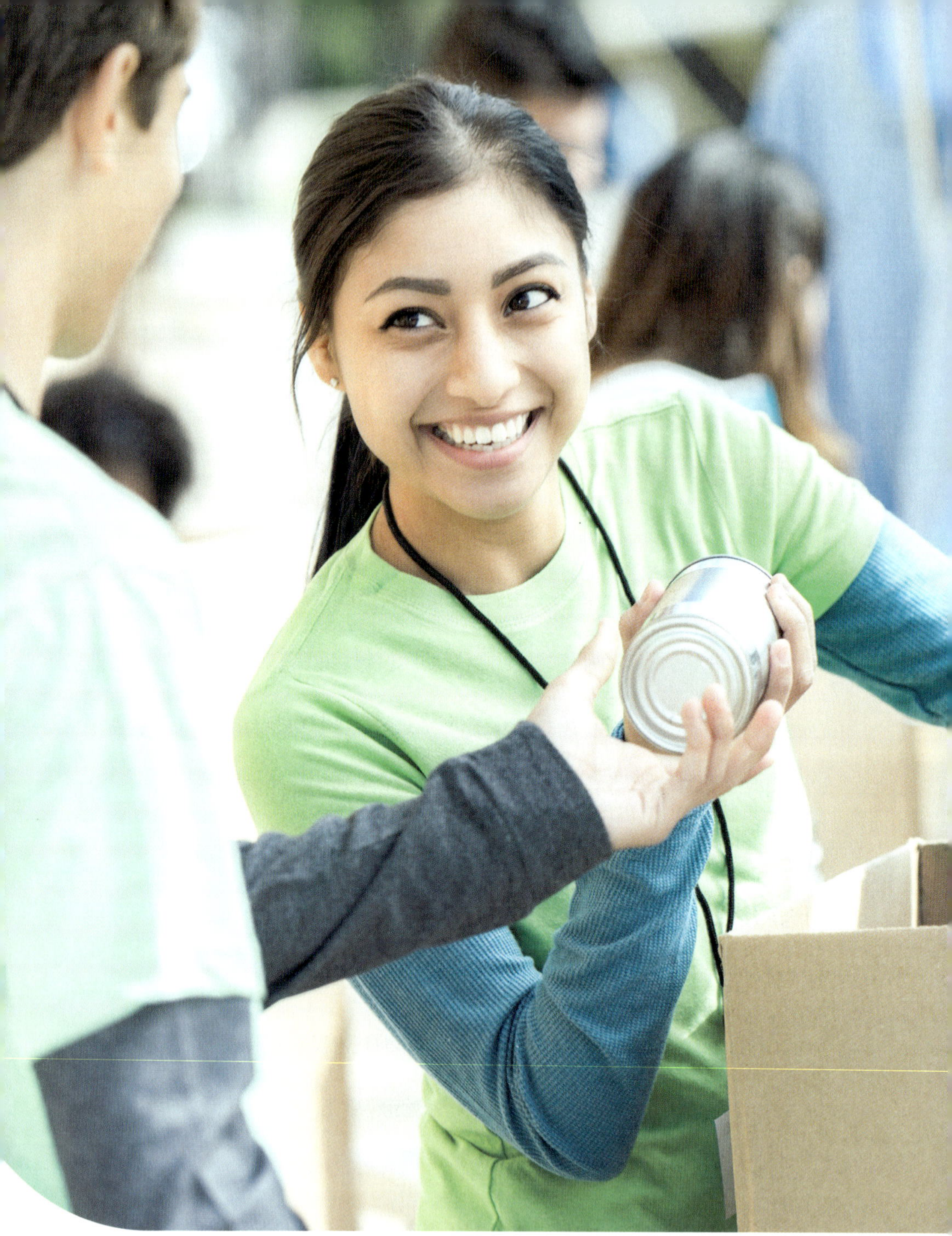

Many people value helping others. They may enjoy volunteering in their free time.

to think good thoughts about themselves and others. They start by wishing themselves happiness. Then they send kind thoughts to someone they love. They might think nice thoughts about someone they don't like, too. Finally, they wish their whole community well.

CHOOSING VALUES

Many people wonder what the meaning of life is. The answer is different for everyone. People have different purposes in life. Family is important to many people. Friends, work, and community are also valuable. For some people, finding purpose is easy. Others take longer to find meaning.

Identifying their values can help people find meaning in life. Values are what people see as most important. Values are what make a person happy, proud, or fulfilled. Knowledge, peace, and adventure are a few examples. People can try writing down their values on a piece of paper. They can think about ways to bring these values into their lives more. If they value knowledge, for

Searching for Meaning

Viktor Frankl was a Jewish psychologist. He survived Nazi concentration camps during World War II (1939–1945). He saw and experienced great suffering. He found that purpose helped people survive the unthinkable. In his book, he identified with a quote attributed to the philosopher Friedrich Nietzsche. It says, "He who has a why to live for can bear with almost any how."

Quoted in Viktor E. Frankl, Man's Search for Meaning. *Washington Square Press, 1963, p. 121.*

example, they could read a new book every month. If they value adventure, they could go on a hike.

Finding purpose, meaning, and spiritual connection in life helps people's well-being. These are also connected to mental and physical health. When a person works on one area of their well-being, all the other areas improve, too. People can do many things to care for themselves every day. These add up to make a healthy life.

GLOSSARY

coordination

the ability of separate parts to work together smoothly

dietician

a medical professional who specializes in nutrition

digestive

relating to the system through which the body absorbs nutrients from food and eliminates waste

meditates

engages in a practice of reflection and focused thought

mental illnesses

medical conditions affecting personality, emotions, or other aspects of the mind

nutritious

having nutrients and other things that support the functioning of the body and mind

resilience

the ability to recover from or adjust to struggle

restrictive

relating to limiting or forbidding something

SOURCE NOTES

INTRODUCTION: VISITING THE DOCTOR

1. Quoted in Sandy Cohen, "How Can You Make 2025 a Healthy New Year? 8 UCLA Health Experts Offer Tips," *UCLA Health*, December 19, 2024. www.uclahealth.org.

CHAPTER ONE: EXERCISE AND NUTRITION

2. Rayven Nairn, "Health at Every Size: A Concept to Reduce Weight-Centric Thinking and to Promote Body Positivity," *Johns Hopkins University*, February 20, 2023. https://wellbeing.jhu.edu.

3. Quoted in "On Teens, Nutrition, and Exercise: How to Encourage Healthy Habits," *Tufts University School of Medicine*, April 9, 2024. https://medicine.tufts.edu.

4. Quoted in Sara Berg, "What Doctors Wish Patients Knew About Sodium Consumption," *American Medical Association*, August 15, 2025. www.ama-assn.org.

CHAPTER TWO: BRAIN HEALTH

5. Kelsey Kidd, "6 Tips to Keep Your Brain Healthy," *Mayo Clinic Health System*, December 29, 2022. www.mayoclinichealthsystem.org.

CHAPTER THREE: MENTAL HEALTH

6. Kristen Neff, *Self-Compassion: The Proven Power of Being Kind to Yourself*. William Morrow, 2025.

CHAPTER FOUR: SOCIAL AND SPIRITUAL WELL-BEING

7. Casper ter Kuile, *The Power of Ritual: Turning Everyday Activities into Soulful Practices*. HarperOne, 2020.

FOR FURTHER RESEARCH

BOOKS

Kate Chynoweth, *Take a Hike!: And Other Ways to De-Stress and Relax in Nature*. Magination Press, 2025.

Marie-Therese Miller, *Developing and Maintaining Relationships*. BrightPoint Press, 2027.

Sheryl Normandeau, *Living with Anxiety*. BrightPoint Press, 2024.

INTERNET SOURCES

"Disability and Mental Health," *YoungMinds*, n.d. www.youngminds.org.uk.

"How to Get Fit and Stay Healthy: Tips for Teens," *HealthyChildren.org*, July 9, 2024. www.healthychildren.org.

Beth C. Long, "Body Image and Self-Esteem," *TeensHealth*, June 2023. http://kidshealth.org.

WEBSITES

Jed Foundation
http://jedfoundation.org

The Jed Foundation offers advice without judgement. The website answers common questions people have about their health.

National Alliance on Mental Illness
www.nami.org/kids-teens-and-young-adults/teens

The National Alliance on Mental Illness (NAMI) has resources for young people to learn about social and emotional well-being. The website also gives tips for people dealing with common mental health struggles.

Self-Care Resources for Young People: Anna Freud
www.annafreud.org

The Anna Freud website provides many resources to support young people. This website includes many practical tips for supporting mental well-being.

INDEX

IMAGE CREDITS

Cover: © Jacek Chabraszewski/Shutterstock Images
5: © VH-Studio/Shutterstock Images
7: © leaf/iStockphoto
9: © Halfpoint/Shutterstock Images
10: © Chalermphon_Tiam/Shutterstock Images
13: © FatCamera/iStockphoto
16: © Quality Stock Arts/Shutterstock Images
19: © Fly View Productions/iStockphoto
20: © SeventyFour/Shutterstock Images
23: © Foto Eak/Shutterstock Images
24: © Imgorthand/iStockphoto
27: © Pressmaster/iStockphoto
29: © Zeynep Demir Aslim/Shutterstock Images
31: © My Life Graphic/Shutterstock Images
32: © PeopleImages/Shutterstock Images
35: © Prostock-Studio/Shutterstock Images
37: © Daniel Hoz/Shutterstock Images
38: © SolStock/iStockphoto
40: © OlgaDykun/Shutterstock Images
45: © True Touch Lifestyle/Shutterstock Images
46: © PeopleImages/Shutterstock Images
49: © Monkey Business Images/Shutterstock Images
51: © SolStock/iStockphoto
53: © SeventyFour/iStockphoto
54: © SDI Productions/iStockphoto

ABOUT THE AUTHOR

Andy Minshew is a writer and book reviewer. He is currently a graduate student at Western Governors University in education technology and instructional design. He loves visiting art museums, participating in his local J.R.R. Tolkien Society branch, and hiking with his family.